Contents

Some words are printed in bold, **like this**. You can find out what they mean in the glossary.

Health and happiness

If you could wish for anything at all, what would it be? Some might wish for possessions, others for wealth or happiness. Many people would put their health first, wishing to be well throughout their lives. We take good health for granted but it is difficult to be happy without being healthy.

The story of Sasha Elterman

In July 1997, Sasha Elterman was a 16-year-old Australian athlete in the best of health. She was selected to represent her country at an international competition in Israel as a swimmer and tennis player. At the opening ceremony, Sasha crossed a makeshift bridge over a badly polluted river to get to the stadium. The bridge collapsed and she fell into the river. Before she was rescued, Sasha swallowed some of the polluted water.

Unfortunately, Sasha had taken in a rare **fungus** infection that made her seriously ill. She was kept in hospital and given just a three percent chance of survival. She underwent more than 30 operations. From being a fit and healthy young woman, illness destroyed her health and her sporting career.

Sasha's story dramatically demonstrates the contrast between good and bad health. You can find out what happened to her on page 21.

"Representing Australia should have been the happiest day of my life. Instead it turned into the worst." [Sasha Elterman, right] →

Why Science Matters

Finding Better Medicines

John Coad

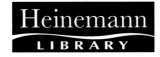

www.heinemannlibrary.co.uk
Visit our website to find out more information about Heinemann Library books.

To order:
☎ Phone +44 (0) 1865 888066
🖷 Fax +44 (0) 1865 314091
🖳 Visit www.heinemannlibrary.co.uk

Heinemann Library is an imprint of **Capstone Global Library Limited**, a company incorporated in England and Wales having its registered office at 7 Pilgrim Street, London, EC4V 6LB – Registered company number: 6695582

Heinemann is a registered trademark of Pearson Education Limited, under licence to Capstone Global Library Limited

Text © Capstone Global Library Limited 2008
First published in hardback in 2008
Paperback edition first published in 2009

Edited by Andrew Farrow, Megan Cotugno, and Harriet Milles
Designed by Steven Mead and Q2A Creative Solutions
Original illustrations © Pearson Education Limited
Illustrated by Gordon Hurden
Picture research by Ruth Blair
Produced by Alison Parsons
Originated by Heinemann Library
Printed and bound in China by Leo Paper Products

ISBN: 978 0 4310 4068 4 (hardback)
12 11 10 09 08
10 9 8 7 6 5 4 3 2 1

ISBN: 978 0 4310 4081 3 (paperback)
13 12 11 10 09
10 9 8 7 6 5 4 3 2 1

British Library Cataloguing in Publication data
Coad, John
Finding better medicines. - (Why science matters)
615.1'0724
A full catalogue record for this book is available from the British Library.

Acknowledgements
We would like to thank the following for permission to reproduce photographs: ©Corbis pp. 10 (Steve Chenn), 33 (Yves Forestier); ©Newspix p. 4; ©Photolibrary.com p. 43 (Pacific Stock); ©Photoshot pp. 6, 31 (UPPA), 26 (Newscom), 30 (Tetra Images), 32 (Talking Sport), 46 (Blend Images), 15, 34, 40, 44; ©Science Photo Library pp. 5 (Mauro Fermariello), 7 (Mark Thomas), 16 (Dr Gopal Murti), 19 (Library of Congress), 21 (John Hadfield), 27 (Sinclair Stammers), 38 (Samuel Ashfield), 39 (Jim Wvinner), 41 (R. Umesh Chandran, TDR, WHO); ©with kind permission of Pfizer Corporate Media Relations, pp. 20, 23, 24, 25. Background images supplied by ©istockphoto.

Cover photograph reproduced with permission of ©Corbis (Firefly Productions). Background image ©istockphoto.

We would like to thank David Ockwell for his invaluable assistance in the preparation of this book.

Every effort has been made to contact copyright holders of any material reproduced in this book. Any omissions will be rectified in subsequent printings if notice is given to the publishers.

Infectious diseases

Organisms that invade our bodies cause infectious diseases. The organisms can be **bacteria**, **viruses**, fungi, or **parasites**. They grow and reproduce inside us and can be passed on to other people. The way in which these organisms make us ill varies. Viruses tend to take over our cells, often destroying them. Some bacteria produce poisonous substances called toxins. Fungi feed off the living material of our bodies.

More than 90 percent of deaths from infectious diseases worldwide are caused by only a handful of diseases – infections of the respiratory system, **AIDS**, diseases that cause diarrhoea, tuberculosis, malaria, and measles.

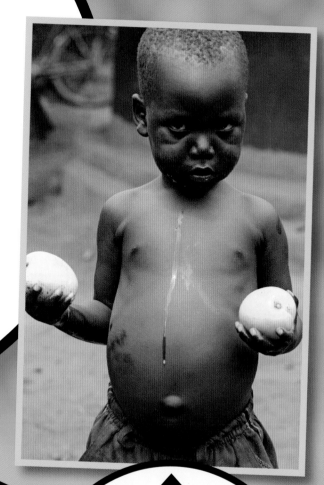

Kwashiorkor is a disease caused by severe protein deficiency in children under five years old. It results in stunted growth, lethargy (lack of energy), diarrhoea, and a swollen abdomen. It is common in less economically developed countries (LEDCs) with a high rate of malnutrition.

Dietary diseases

What we eat or drink – or do not eat and drink – can make us ill. Too much fatty food can cause obesity, heart disease, and diabetes. Too much alcohol can lead to liver damage and heart disease. Scientists are even exploring the possibility that some foods can cause cancer.

If we don't eat enough of what our body needs, we become ill. For example, our bodies need vitamins from our food. Without vitamin C we develop a skin disease called scurvy. A shortage of vitamin D in children leads to a bone disease called rickets. It is easy to avoid such diseases by eating a balanced diet.

Stephen Hawking

One of the world's greatest living scientists, Professor Stephen Hawking (born 1942), has done much to advance our understanding of the universe. However just as remarkable as his scientific discoveries is his fight – and survival – against a crippling degenerative (gradually worsening) disease. He suffers from motor neurone disease, also called ALS. This disease involves a degeneration of the nervous system, which leads to wasting away of muscles. Eventually it results in complete paralysis. There is no effective treatment for this disease.

↑ With advanced motor neurone disease, Stephen Hawking is confined to a wheelchair. A specially designed computer acts as a voice simulator, allowing him to talk.

Inherited diseases

Some diseases are passed on from parents to their children in their **genes**. These are inherited diseases. One of the most common inherited diseases in northern Europe is cystic fibrosis. Around one in twenty-five people of northern European descent carry a faulty gene in their **DNA** that could cause cystic fibrosis. Both parents must carry the gene for the baby to inherit the disease.

Cystic fibrosis affects the lungs. Normal lungs produce a fluid designed to trap dust particles that are breathed in. The liquid is easily cleared from the lungs. In cystic fibrosis patients, the liquid is thicker. It is not cleared from the lungs and tends to block the airways. This leads to coughing to try and clear it. Like all genetic diseases there is no cure.

A pill when we're ill?

What do we do when we are ill? We have a number of options.

- Ignore it and hope to get better. This often works. The human body has a remarkable ability to repair itself. Our **immune system** wins against most common infections.

- Go to a pharmacy and buy a medicine. Treatments bought in this way are called over-the-counter medicines. They are generally safe. However, to cure ourselves in this way, we must get the diagnosis right.

- Visit a doctor. We might then be prescribed a more powerful medicine. The doctor will check that we are suitable to take the medicine. Prescription-only medicines must be taken in the right doses and only by the person they are prescribed for.

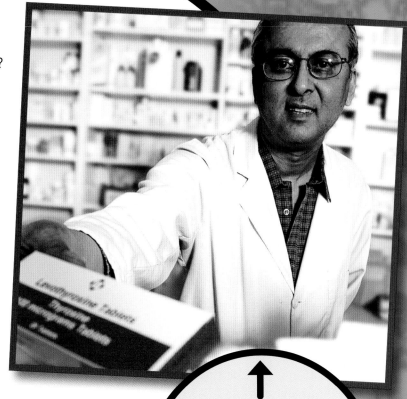

We can buy many over-the-counter medicines from pharmacies. This book is mainly concerned with prescription-only medicines that we can only obtain from doctors.

IN YOUR HOME: THE MEDICINE CUPBOARD

Around most homes there are leftover pills, powders, creams, and lotions which we no longer use. Medicines that are out-of-date or are taken by the wrong people can be dangerous. Each year hundreds of children are admitted to hospitals for treatment after wrongly taking medicines. If we are given prescription medicines, it is important that we finish the course of treatment. Any unfinished medicines should be returned to the pharmacy. Medicine cupboards should always be kept locked and out of the reach of children.

Simple medicines for treating indigestion

Indigestion is easy to identify and treat. If you eat rich food or eat too quickly you might feel indigestion as a burning sensation in the stomach. Sometimes it is felt higher up in the chest and is known as heartburn. The medical term for indigestion is dyspepsia.

The stomach produces a strong acid that helps digest food and protects you against infection. A layer of mucus lines the stomach and acts as a barrier against the acid. If the acid gets too strong or the mucus layer is damaged then the acid irritates the lining – it begins to digest the stomach wall!

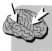

THE SCIENCE YOU LEARN: ACIDS AND BASES

Most indigestion tablets contain chemicals that will neutralize the acid in the stomach. The opposite of an acid is a base. The chemicals in most indigestion tablets are bases.

The strength of an acid is measured on the pH scale. Strong acids have a low pH value of 1 or 2. A very weak acid is pH 6, and pH 7 is neutral. If bases dissolve in water they make alkalis. Alkalis have pH values higher than 7.

In some cases stomach acid rises up the oesophagus. The diagram shows that the pain will be quite high in the chest just behind the breastbone (sternum). Many people with chest pains have wrongly thought they were having a heart attack when it was just heartburn.

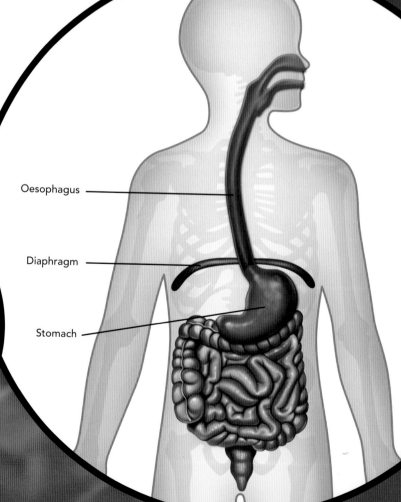

Oesophagus

Diaphragm

Stomach

Indigestion tablets

Several bases are used in indigestion tablets. The simplest and most common is sodium bicarbonate ($NaHCO_3$). It reacts with stomach acid to make carbon dioxide gas. After the pain is relieved you might burp.

Calcium carbonate (chalk, $CaCO_3$), aluminium hydroxide ($Al(OH)_3$), magnesium hydroxide ($Mg(OH)_2$), and magnesium carbonate ($MgCO_3$) are all bases. Some tablets have a combination of these chemicals.

Other indigestion medicines contain a chemical that lines the stomach walls. The lining protects the stomach from the acid. Alternatively doctors can prescribe pills that stop the stomach making acid.

INVESTIGATION: WHICH INDIGESTION TABLETS NEUTRALIZE THE MOST ACID?

This is an investigation you can easily carry out in your school laboratory. You will need to choose an acid. The acid in the stomach is hydrochloric acid and is similar in strength to the acid available in your school laboratory. Such an acid should only be used in a laboratory under supervision from a trained science teacher.

Equipment

indigestion tablets	mortar and pestle
glass rod	pipette
beaker	pH paper
dilute hydrochloric acid	

Procedure

1. Crush an indigestion tablet using the mortar and pestle and put it in a beaker.
2. Using a dropping pipette, add several drops of acid.
3. Stir well then use pH paper to check the pH of the mixture. The tablet will have neutralized the acid, so the pH should be 7.
4. Continue to add drops of acid, stir well each time, and check the pH. Keep going until the pH drops to low values. The tablet can now no longer neutralize the acid.
5. Repeat Steps 1–4 with other makes of indigestion tablet. Each time you will find out how many drops of acid one tablet will neutralize.
6. How could you make the investigation more accurate? Could you measure the volume of acid rather than counting drops?

Pain, pills, and potions

One of the greatest medical needs has always been to reduce pain. An Egyptian papyrus from 1500 BC prescribed myrtle leaves for stomach pain. Hippocrates, a famous ancient Greek doctor, made juice from willow bark to relieve pain and fever 2,000 years ago. Today, although there are drugs to treat aches and pains, they do not work for everyone and some are highly addictive. Scientists are continually searching for better treatments.

THE SCIENCE YOU LEARN: HOW DO WE FEEL PAIN?

Pain is a defence mechanism for the body. Damaging part of the body causes an unpleasant sensation that warns us not to do the same again. A pain is usually a message that something is wrong. Nerves near damaged cells send signals to the spinal cord, and on to the brain. The brain interprets and acts on the message.

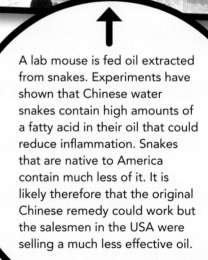

A lab mouse is fed oil extracted from snakes. Experiments have shown that Chinese water snakes contain high amounts of a fatty acid in their oil that could reduce inflammation. Snakes that are native to America contain much less of it. It is likely therefore that the original Chinese remedy could work but the salesmen in the USA were selling a much less effective oil.

Snake oil salesmen

In the 19th century, salesmen travelled the United States selling treatments for numerous ailments. The salesman often had an assistant who would cry out that the medicine being advertised had cured all his ailments.

A common cure-all was snake oil. This had been a remedy in China for aches and pains, and was brought to the United States by Chinese railway workers. The salesmen were con-men and the remedy did not work.

The world's best seller

It has long been known that chewing willow bark can relieve pain. In 1838, Italian chemist Raffaele Piria (1814–65) extracted and purified the chemical in the bark that actually provides the relief. He named it salicylic acid. Twenty years later, a company in Germany was set up to manufacture salicylic acid. It was easy and inexpensive to make. One drawback was that salicylic acid had a very bitter taste. Chemists modified it, creating a new compound that they called aspirin.

IN YOUR HOME: ASPIRIN

Injured cells make chemicals called **prostaglandins**. These activate our nerves, sending pain messages to the brain. **Enzymes** called **cyclooxygenases** (COX) help make the prostaglandins. Aspirin sticks to cyclooxygenases and stops them working. Therefore no prostaglandins are made and the pain is less severe.

THE SCIENCE YOU LEARN:
PROTEINS AND ENZYMES

Our bodies contain **proteins** – huge molecules with hundreds of atoms bonded together. They are an essential part of body tissue and are also needed for the growth and repair of cells. Enzymes are a type of protein that help chemical processes take place inside our cells. Without enzymes the reactions in our body would be very slow or would not occur at all. Each enzyme is very specific and speeds up just one reaction. Each has a special shape with a region we call the active site. Reacting molecules bind onto the active site and the reaction takes place. A drug molecule can bind to an active site, preventing the enzyme from doing its job.

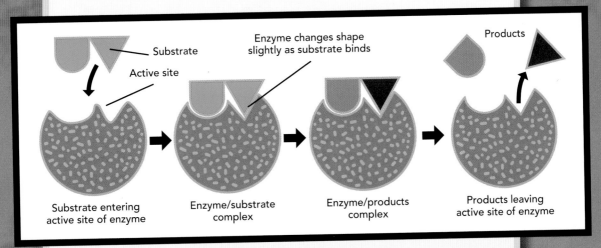

Substrate

Active site

Enzyme changes shape slightly as substrate binds

Products

Substrate entering active site of enzyme

Enzyme/substrate complex

Enzyme/products complex

Products leaving active site of enzyme

Side effects

Aspirin is a popular and useful drug but it does have faults. Some people are allergic to it. It also has a dangerous **side effect**.

The trouble is that aspirin works on all cyclooxygenase (COX) enzymes – not just the one at the injury site. In the stomach, prostaglandins help keep the lining thick. Aspirin interferes with their production and the lining thins. This allows acids to irritate the stomach. Aspirin can cause bleeding in the stomach and a large dose can kill. On the other hand, aspirin can stop blood clotting. This helps people at risk of heart attacks or strokes because these conditions are caused by blood clots.

The molecular structure of aspirin

Drugs like aspirin are described as small molecules. An aspirin molecule might seem complicated but it is small compared to the huge structure of a protein.

Other common treatments

There are other medicines that are used to treat pain. Some can be bought freely, others require a prescription. Ibuprofen and paracetamol are common over-the-counter medicines that reduce moderate pain and inflammation. Ibuprofen works in a similar way to aspirin but has less severe side effects. Paracetamol (also called acetaminophen) works slightly differently. It blocks the formation of prostaglandins in the brain instead of at the source of pain. How it does this is not fully understood.

Although these painkillers are readily available in pharmacies it must be remembered that they are potentially dangerous drugs. An overdose of any of them can kill.

Treating severe pain

A milky liquid extracted from poppy seeds has been used as a powerful painkiller for thousands of years. This extract is opium and it contains a chemical called morphine. Morphine sticks to a particular type of protein in the brain called an opiate **receptor**. It blocks pain signals to the brain. Although opiates are effective, they are dangerously addictive. The body also gets used to them so larger and larger doses are needed to block the same amount of pain. Very high doses of opiates are fatal. Scientists are continually trying to find new treatments for severe pain.

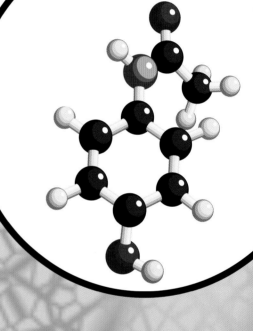

The molecular structure of paracetamol

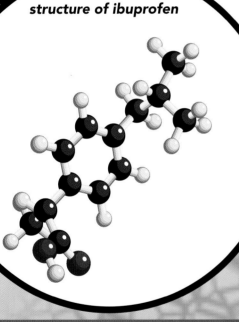

The molecular structure of ibuprofen

CUTTING EDGE: COX-2 INHIBITORS

Scientists discovered that the COX enzyme in the stomach is slightly different from the one responsible for pain. Researchers rushed to find new drugs that would not harm the stomach. A new family of painkillers was developed called COX-2 inhibitors. Two were introduced in 1999 and quickly became best-selling drugs with millions of prescriptions issued each year. The new painkillers were particularly effective for patients with painful arthritis. All seemed well until the new COX-2 inhibitors were shown to have potentially dangerous side effects.

Bugs and wonder drugs

Bacteria are minute living organisms that can only be seen under a powerful microscope. They live almost everywhere on our planet and are vital in maintaining living systems. They decompose waste, trap nitrogen from the air for plants to use, and form part of the food chain. Millions of bacteria live inside you helping to digest fibre from fruit and vegetables. They even manufacture some vitamins in your body.

However, some bacteria are very harmful. If they get inside your body the conditions are perfect (warm and moist with plenty of food) for them to multiply rapidly. They release poisons called toxins. In the past, people often died as a result of infected minor injuries. Today most infections can be cured easily.

BACTERIAL DISEASES		
Disease	**Region affected**	**Bacterium**
Sore throat, tonsilitis	Respiratory system – ear, nose, and throat	*Streptococcus pyogenes*
Whooping cough	Respiratory system	*Bordetella pertussis*
Tuberculosis	The lungs – sometimes other areas, e.g. brain, bones, kidneys	*Mycobacterium tuberculosis*
Food poisoning	Digestive system	*Escherichia coli*
Cholera	Gut, particularly the bowel	*Vibrio cholerae*
Meningitis	Brain and spinal cord	*Haemophilus influenzae*
Leprosy	Nervous system and skin	*Mycobacterium leprae*
Syphilis	Sexual organs	*Treponema pallidum*
Tetanus	Nervous system	*Clostridium tetani*

The first antibiotic

In 1928, British scientist Alexander Fleming (1881–1955) was studying some harmful bacteria. He grew visible colonies of millions of bacteria on petri dishes. One dish became contaminated with mould and he noticed something unusual. Where the mould grew, there were no bacteria. Fleming grew the mould and made a liquid extract that killed many types of dangerous bacteria. He called his discovery penicillin – the first **antibiotic**.

Ten years later, Australian scientist Howard Florey (1898–1968) and Ernst Chain (1906–1979), originally from Berlin, decided to do more experiments with penicillin. Progress was slow but in 1940 they finally managed to extract 0.1 g of penicillin.

The first patient was treated in 1941. A policeman who had cut himself shaving had developed a life-threatening infection. Florey and Chain treated him with penicillin. Within 24 hours the patient showed signs of recovery! Unfortunately the supplies of penicillin ran out, and the policeman had a relapse and died.

Research into penicillin moved to the United States. With a new strain of mould and by adapting the equipment, large quantities of penicillin were made. By 1944, there was enough to treat war casualties and thousands of lives were saved.

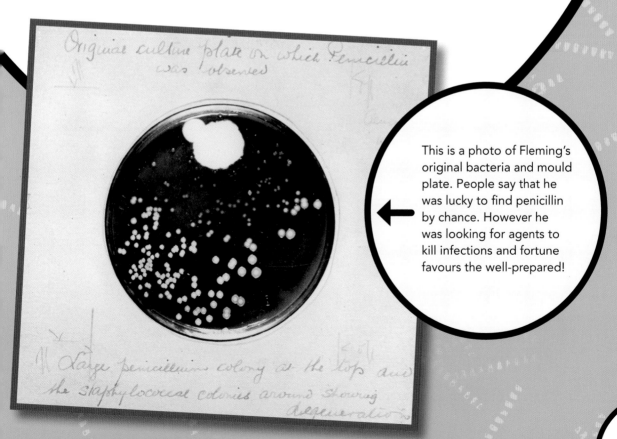

This is a photo of Fleming's original bacteria and mould plate. People say that he was lucky to find penicillin by chance. However he was looking for agents to kill infections and fortune favours the well-prepared!

THE SCIENCE YOU LEARN: THE IMMUNE SYSTEM

Our bodies have amazing defences against infection. The skin acts as a barrier to infection, while tears and saliva contain an enzyme that kills bacteria. When organisms do manage to enter the bloodstream, our defences spring into action. The immune system involves white blood cells. One type of white blood cell, called a **macrophage**, engulfs and destroys bacteria, and viruses.

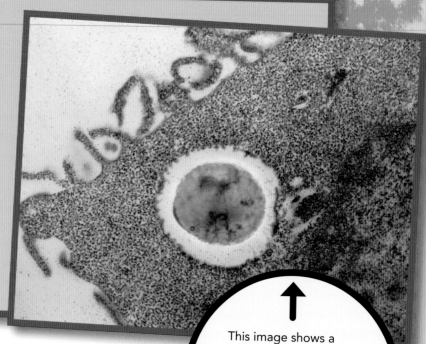

This image shows a macrophage engulfing a harmful bacteria (coloured blue). Marcrophages are a vital part of the immune system.

Antibiotics at work

Bacteria link molecules together into a tough barrier which becomes their cell wall. Penicillin is similar to one of the molecules used to make this barrier. As the bacterium grows it uses penicillin along with its usual molecules. This weakens the cell wall and eventually it bursts apart. Other antibiotics stop bacteria reproducing, and some stop them producing proteins.

Since the discovery of penicillin, thousands of other antibiotics have been developed. Bacteria called *Streptomyces* were found to produce antibiotics. Chemists began to alter the antibiotic molecules to make them stay in the body longer and be more effective. However, one problem with antibiotics is that they also kill good bacteria.

 THE SCIENCE YOU LEARN: SUPERBUGS

A bacterium called *Staphylococcus aureus* is found in the respiratory system of many people. In most cases it is harmless. However, it has mutated and a variation of it has developed a resistance to antibiotics such as penicillin and methicillin. This methicillin-resistant *Staphylococcus aureus* is now called MRSA. It is exceedingly difficult to treat and is often referred to as a superbug.

Bacteria fight back

Bacteria can change to resist antibiotics. Sometimes the DNA in a bacterium will mutate (change) so that it makes different proteins. This might alter the bacterium so the antibiotics don't work. All offspring of that mutated bacterium will also be resistant. This means that we must be careful how we use antibiotics. If we do not finish the course of treatment given by a doctor, any bacteria not killed will be the stronger, more resistant ones. They will reproduce which will lead to even more resistance.

Viruses

In 1892, Russian botanist Dmitri Ivanovsky (1864–1920) was investigating diseased tobacco plants. He made an extract from the plants and passed it through a fine filter that would remove any bacteria. He found that the liquid could still transmit the disease to healthy tobacco plants. Clearly there was an infectious agent smaller than bacteria. The name virus (which means poison in Latin) was used to describe these agents.

Viruses are parasites. Outside a cell they are lifeless but when they invade a cell they take over the cell mechanisms to make more viruses. They usually destroy the cell in the process. The common cold is caused by a virus. Many virus infections are much more serious. Influenza, measles, German measles, mumps, smallpox, polio, hepatitis, herpes, and AIDS are all caused by viruses which are fairly easily passed from one person to another.

 CUTTING EDGE: ACYCLOVIR

Herpes viruses cause diseases like chicken pox, shingles, and cold sores. A herpes virus gets into a human cell, takes over the nucleus (central part), and makes thousands more viruses. Acyclovir is a drug that can pass into the nucleus and is similar to a chemical used to make DNA. The virus uses the acyclovir in new DNA but once it is used, the DNA chain cannot be lengthened and no more virus can be made.

The AIDS epidemic

AIDS was first recognized and named in the early 1980s. It is caused by HIV (human immunodeficiency virus). The virus invades white blood cells where it reproduces. It destroys the cells that are a vital part of our immune system. The body can no longer fight off routine infections and it is these infections that finally lead to death. The virus is spread by sexual contact or through infected blood. About 36 million people around the world are infected with HIV.

Vaccines

It is very difficult to find drugs that work against viruses. Attacking the virus will also attack the infected cells. One way of protecting against some viral infections is through vaccinations.

CASE STUDY

"I thought I had made a mistake"

In the 1980s, AIDS was spreading rapidly. There was no medicine to treat it. In 1984 an American scientist, Marty St Clair, who was working for a major pharmaceutical company, made an important discovery. She had been carrying out tests in her laboratory in which she put live cells into 350 petri dishes then added the virus. A series of different potential drugs were then put into the dishes. If the drug did not work, the virus would destroy the cells and there would be a gap in the layer of cells. Marty St Clair had to examine every dish and count every gap.

"I was holding them up to the window," she said. "I came to 16 dishes, none of which had any gaps." All were labelled as containing a compound called AZT. "I rang my supervisor, then I thought: 'I wonder if I forgot to put the virus in these 16?'" Fortunately, Marty St Clair had not made a mistake. She had found the first ever medicine to treat HIV.

Antigens and antibodies

Your immune system recognizes strange cells that enter your body. Every cell has unique chemicals on its surface called **antigens**. Your immune system recognizes that the antigens on invading microorganisms are different to the ones on your own cells. It then makes chemicals called **antibodies**. The antibodies stick to the antigens, destroying or inactivating the cell. Once the microorganisms are out of action, they are engulfed by macrophage cells.

The first time you meet a new microorganism, you get ill. There is a delay while your body makes the right antibody. The next time you meet the microorganism, the white blood cells can start making the right antibody straight away. This means you destroy the invaders before they have time to make you feel ill. You are immune to the disease.

When you are given a **vaccine** made of weakened or dead microorganisms, your body has the chance to develop the right antibodies against the disease. Then if you meet the real disease, you will already have the right antibodies in place and will be protected against the disease.

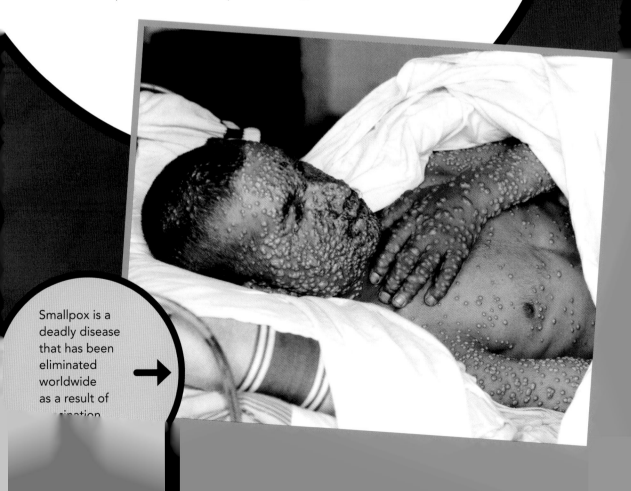

Smallpox is a deadly disease that has been eliminated worldwide as a result of

Vaccine success

Polio (poliomyelitis) is a disease that affects the nervous system and leads to muscle paralysis. When the muscles controlling breathing are paralyzed, death is likely. Polio is highly infectious and was untreatable until scientists found vaccines that would work. Two different vaccines were produced.

One vaccine was made by growing the virus then killing it. Dead virus was injected into volunteers. The antigens on dead viruses trigger the immune system to create antibodies. An alternative vaccine used a weakened strain of the polio virus that would give children immunity without them getting the disease.

Vaccinations against polio have been carried out since the 1960s. From being a terrifying disease that crippled millions, polio has been almost eliminated. There were just 2,000 cases worldwide in 2006 compared to 350,000 in 1968.

The British Government launched a huge publicity campaign in the 1960s to persuade people to be vaccinated against polio. The poster campaign was very important. Few people had TV, and there was no Internet or email to spread the message.

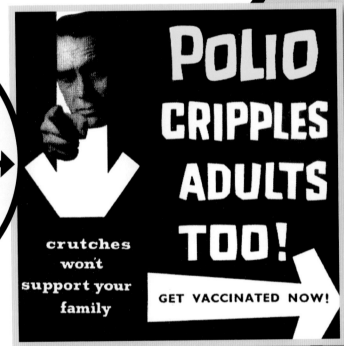

POLIO CRIPPLES ADULTS TOO!

crutches won't support your family

GET VACCINATED NOW!

Vaccine failure

In April 1984, the United States' Health and Human Service Secretary gave a speech about AIDS and announced: "We hope to have a vaccine [against AIDS] ready for testing in about two years. Yet another terrible disease is about to yield to patience, persistence, and outright genius." Sadly that proved wildly inaccurate. So far, all attempts to find a vaccine for HIV/AIDS have failed.

Fungal infections

Fungi are microorganisms. There are over 50 known fungal diseases, including athlete's foot, ringworm, and thrush. Fungi grow on the skin or in a moist, warm area such as the mouth or genitals. Developing medicines to kill fungal infections is difficult because the cells of fungi are very similar to human cells. There are slight differences that scientists have to target in order to kill the fungi and not the human cells.

What happened to Sasha?

As we read on page 4, healthy athlete Sasha Elterman caught the rare fungus *P. boydii* and was treated with antifungal medicines. The drugs were not effective and three times her doctors expected her to die. Then her medical team heard of a new antifungal drug called voriconazole. The drug was new and no one knew if it was safe or would work. However, Sasha had nothing to lose. Supplies were flown to her and amazingly she showed an almost immediate improvement. After extensive treatment with the drug, Sasha recovered. In the year 2000 she ran with the Olympic torch at the start of the Sydney games.

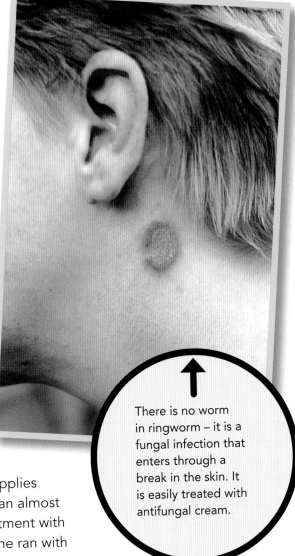

There is no worm in ringworm – it is a fungal infection that enters through a break in the skin. It is easily treated with antifungal cream.

THE SCIENCE YOU LEARN: OPPORTUNISTIC INFECTIONS

There are more bacteria on your body than there are cells in it! Some of these bacteria are helpful to us and most do us no harm. Our bacteria have adapted to their environments, and created a delicate balance. If this balance is upset there is more opportunity for other organisms to move in. The balance can be upset when we use antibiotics or if the immune system is weakened. Fungi are quick to seize upon such opportunities and many fungal infections occur in this way.

Drug discovery

This chapter focuses on a drug called maraviroc that was developed as a treatment for AIDS. This story illustrates the difficult and expensive process of drug discovery that pharmaceutical companies use to create new medicines.

Pharmaceutical companies research many diseases. To treat a particular disease, their scientists must find out what goes wrong in the body, then come up with an idea to tackle it. They need to change how one of the body's biological processes works. The part of the process they need to affect is called the target.

In 1996, scientists discovered how HIV gets into white blood cells. The virus sticks onto a protein on the cell surface before joining with the cell membrane and entering the cell. Scientists realized that if a compound could be found to bind to the protein, the virus would not be able to enter the cell. It would not be able to reproduce and destroy the cell. The race was on to find a suitable compound.

Screening

The next step is to find a chemical that will have the desired effect on the target. One way of doing this is through screening. Pharmaceutical companies can have millions of stored compounds. Their scientists devise experiments to test the compounds on the biological target. Robots carry out the testing. Finding a suitable compound is largely a matter of chance.

CUTTING EDGE: COMPUTATIONAL CHEMISTRY

Modern computer technology can be used instead of screening to find a compound. Kate Brown, a British scientist, is a computational chemist. She uses software to create virtual molecules to study their structures and how they might interact with proteins. She can examine the structure of enzymes and design a drug to fit into the active site. She must then work out whether it will stick there. Kate works closely with other skilled chemists who determine the structures of proteins using X-rays.

Maraviroc – screening

The pharmaceutical company, Pfizer, was involved in the search. Pfizer chemists had a million compounds to test, and eventually found five that would bind weakly to the protein on the cell surface. They chose the one that stuck best as their starting point for further research.

Maraviroc – getting the candidate

Chemists take the starting compound and try to improve on it. Pfizer chemists spent nearly three years changing atoms and groups of atoms in the compound to make it work better. Several promising molecules that stuck well to the protein were rejected for other reasons. One interfered with the working of the heart. Another damaged the liver, and another would not go through the gut wall into the bloodstream. Eventually, after making nearly 1,000 new compounds, they found one that worked well. Their job was over – they had their **drug candidate**.

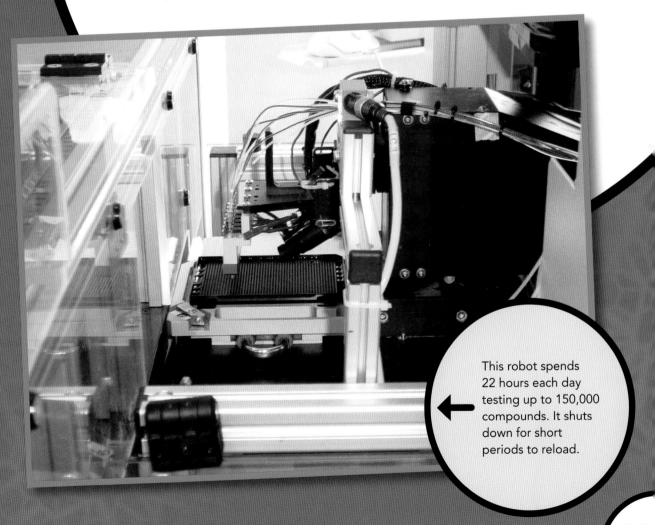

This robot spends 22 hours each day testing up to 150,000 compounds. It shuts down for short periods to reload.

Maraviroc – development

The drug candidate had to be tested in many ways. Would it be safe? How would it keep in different climates? What should it be mixed with to make a pill, and what dose would patients take?

Chemists found ways of making maraviroc on a larger scale. They found out about its **solubility**. This was important as they needed to know how it would dissolve and move around in the blood. They also found out what it could be mixed with. They simulated different climates and looked at how it kept in those conditions. Eventually they made pills to give to people.

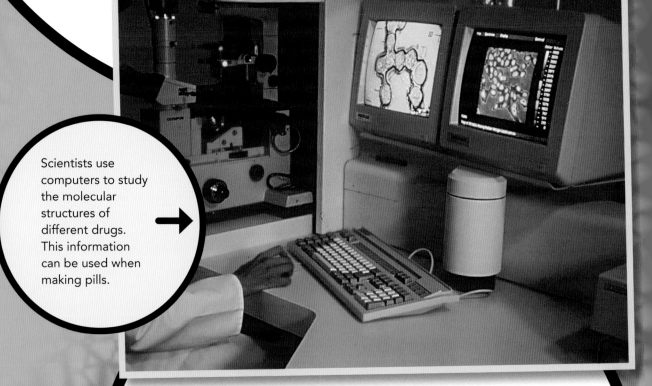

Scientists use computers to study the molecular structures of different drugs. This information can be used when making pills.

The right formulation

When you take a pill, you are not taking the pure drug. Other substances are mixed in. These might be sweeteners, preservatives, fillers that bulk up the tablet, and binders that hold it all together. Sometimes chemicals are added to stop the contents sticking to the pill-making machines. Other chemicals make the pill disperse in your stomach. Formulation scientists find the best mixture of ingredients and test the pills.

INVESTIGATION PANEL: TESTING MEDICINES

Medicines are tested to prove that they work and are safe. Scientists also want to vary the dose given to a patient to see what works best. School science tells us we must repeat experiments to get reliable results.

Also, for a test to be fair, only one factor (called the independent variable) must change in order to see what effect it has. Everything else must be kept constant.

Scientists change the independent variable – the dose of medicine. They then measure the dependent variable – what happens to the patient.

However, testing a drug needs to be carried out on more than just one patient. Once we start changing the person as well, we no longer have a simple fair test. Every person is different and can be affected differently by a drug. Therefore, a different style of investigation has to be carried out in which lots of people are tested.

People's behaviour might also change if they think they are being treated with a medicine. They might begin to feel better just at the thought! For this reason, a dummy medicine – called a **placebo** – is given to some patients.

The placebo looks and tastes exactly like the real medicine, and the patients do not know whether they have the placebo or the real thing.

Doctors might also observe a patient differently if they know he or she is receiving a medicine. They might want the medicine to work and look harder for signs of improvement. For this reason, the doctors often do not know who is receiving the placebo. Trials like this are called double blind trials because neither the patient nor the doctor know who is having the real medicine.

Finding the best mixture of components in a pill is a painstaking process. Here a scientist uses a tablet analysis machine to test whether all the substances in the pill will stick together well enough.

Maraviroc – phase 1 trials

Before being given to humans, maraviroc was tested in dogs and rats. Tests on humans are called **clinical trials**. The drug is first given to a small number of healthy volunteers. The purpose is to find out what the human body does to the drug – how the body digests it, how long it lasts in the body, and how it is excreted (removed). Scientists also want to find out if there are any obvious side effects. The volunteers start on a very low dose, which is increased over time if all goes well. The phase 1 trial showed scientists that maraviroc was safe and was absorbed well into the bloodstream.

Maraviroc – further trials

If a drug is successful at phase 1 trials, it moves to phase 2. Usually a few hundred real patients are treated with the drug. To pass the phase 2 testing, the medicine must work better than existing therapies, and there must be no serious side effects. Pfizer scientists were delighted with the maraviroc phase 2 results. Patients treated with the drug showed a 90 percent reduction in the amount of virus in their blood after just two weeks, and there were no serious side effects.

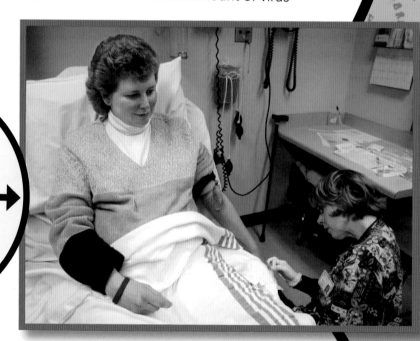

A volunteer has a blood sample taken. Doctors can then see how much of the drug is in the bloodstream and work out how long it lasts in the body.

Maraviroc – big decisions

A pharmaceutical company must decide whether to continue trials after phase 2. That is because there has to be a bigger, much more expensive phase 3 clinical trial.

Phase 3 trials are designed to show that the drug works and is safe. Thousands of volunteer patients are monitored by doctors to check the medicine works, and identify problems that arise from long-term use. Results of the trials determine the dosage for patients and how doctors are instructed to use the drug.

Another company developing a rival to maraviroc withdrew its drug when it caused liver damage in patients. As maraviroc's phase 3 trial continued, one patient also developed severe liver problems. There were fears that maraviroc too would fail until it was shown that other medicines were probably causing the liver problems. Maraviroc came through the phase 3 trials and the results confirmed that it did work by reducing the virus in HIV-infected patients.

These fluorescent light micrographs of human white blood cells show a negative (left) and positive (right) result for the disease HIV. The cells that show up green indicate a negative result.

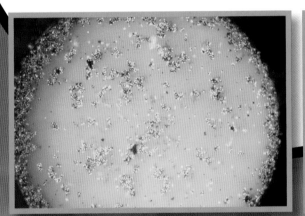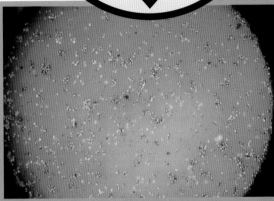

CASE STUDY

A phase 1 disaster

In 2006, eight healthy young men volunteered to take part in a phase 1 clinical trial at Northwick Park Hospital in London. Six men were given a drug called a **monoclonal antibody**. Within a short period of time, all six men were admitted to intensive care. Two of them were in a critical condition with multiple organ failure. The men lived, but they have been damaged for life. The company carrying out the test was criticized for the way it conducted the trial and further work on the drug was abandoned.

Maraviroc – submission and approval

New medicines are very tightly controlled. Pharmaceutical companies must submit all their findings from clinical trials, along with all the details of how they make the drug, to government agencies. In the United States, this is the Food and Drug Administration (FDA). In Europe, it is the European Medicines Agency (EMEA), and in Australia it is the Therapeutic Goods Agency (TGA). Before a new drug can be marketed it must, by law, be approved by these agencies.

Results of maraviroc's clinical trials and all other relevant information were submitted to the FDA and EMEA in 2006. Approval always takes a long time but the FDA sped up the process given the need for a new HIV/AIDS drug. Maraviroc was approved by both agencies in the summer of 2007. Once it was approved, doctors were given guidance on which patients it should be prescribed to.

SCIENCE IN YOUR HOME:
INFORMATION IN THE PACKET

Inside a pill packet there will also be an information leaflet. The leaflet outlines what the scientists have found out during the clinical trials. It will tell you all about the drug, any side effects, dosage information, what the medicine must not be taken with, and when not to take the medicine.

The trials go on

Even when a drug is approved, it is still on trial. There is a chance that unexpected problems will arise. Doctors who find that a patient appears to have been badly affected by a drug can report it. Data is collected and if necessary the information in the packet will be changed. Very occasionally, the use of the drug may become restricted.

How much does it all cost?

Discovering and developing a new drug is an expensive business. Costs are usually quoted in United States dollars (U.S. $). The current estimate is between U.S. $800 million and U.S. $1.2 billion for one drug. If the drug sells well, pharmaceutical companies can get that money back and make a good profit.

What is to stop another company copying the drug and selling it much more cheaply? The answer is a **patent**. A pharmaceutical company must show that a product is completely new, involves an inventive step, is not obvious, and is useful. The product can then be patented. This protects the product from being copied for 20 years. In that time, the company can get back the money it invested and make a profit.

When the 20 years end, anyone can copy the drug. It is then known as a **generic** medicine. Companies that have not had to invest in the research and development will make it and sell it cheaply. Patents arouse strong feelings on both sides.

Without patents there will be no new medicines.

Patents ensure companies can recoup the huge sums invested in research.

A patent gives a company the power to charge what it likes.

Patents make new medicines unaffordable for poor countries.

Safety and side effects

A perfect drug would only affect the part of the biological process involved with the disease. Unfortunately this rarely happens. Drugs are often designed to bind to a protein in the body to stop it doing its normal job. As proteins come in families, a drug that binds to one protein in a family may also bind to another similar one. This will cause unwanted changes in the body that we call side effects. Proteins are involved in many processes around the body so a drug may act where its effects are not needed, again causing side effects.

Every drug has side effects. Even simple drugs such as aspirin have unwanted side effects. Often, all possible side effects are not apparent until many people have tried the drug for some time. Side effects might be as simple as increased thirst or weight gain. More seriously, the drug could affect the nervous system leading to depression. Sometimes the side effects are quite peculiar.

- A 78-year-old man using an antifungal medicine began to hear music in his head. He even compiled a list of the song titles he heard. When doctors changed his medicine, the music stopped
- Patients using a drug to treat Parkinson's disease turned into compulsive gamblers. One woman lost U.S. $100,000!

IN YOUR HOME: GRAPEFRUIT GIVES AN ADDED PUNCH

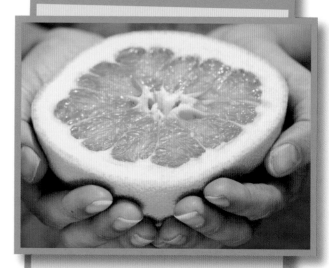

Felodipine is a drug designed to treat tension and lower blood pressure. When it was being trialled, volunteers who also drank grapefruit juice showed unexpected side effects. Their symptoms included dizziness, facial flushing, headaches, and rapid heartbeats. Researchers worked out the problem. There is an enzyme in the body that naturally breaks down the felodipine. Grapefruit juice contains a chemical that blocks this enzyme. Therefore the drug is not removed from the body and it is much more effective. Grapefruit juice doubled the drug's effect on blood pressure and heart rate.

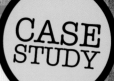

Thalidomide

In 1953, a new drug was discovered in Germany. Within four years it was on the market and being hailed as a wonder treatment for insomnia (sleeplessness), coughs, colds, and headaches. It was called thalidomide. Many doctors prescribed it to pregnant women who were suffering from morning sickness. It did relieve the sickness but had a terrible side effect. In 1961, a doctor noticed a sudden increase in the number of babies born with deformities. All of the babies' mothers had been taking thalidomide.

By the time the drug was withdrawn from use, 10,000 babies had been born with deformities. The worst affected of them died but many survived and are still alive today.

Thalidomide affected the development of the **foetus** during early pregnancy. Limbs failed to develop properly and many babies were born with short flipper-like arms and legs, and reduced numbers of fingers. In some foetuses, internal organs were also affected.

Thalidomide stops blood vessels growing in the limbs of developing foetuses. Recently scientists decided to test the drug again to see if it could stop cancer from growing by blocking blood vessel development.

Risks and benefits

People take risks all the time. Crossing the road, driving a car, even playing sport can lead to injury or worse. We choose to do things where the risk is low and the benefit is high. Taking medicines is similar. There are risks in taking them but we usually judge that the benefits outweigh the risks.

Adverse drug reactions (ADRs)

Many people are admitted to hospital each year as a result of harmful reactions to medicines. In the United States, the number of bad reactions nearly tripled between 1998 and 2005. There are now more than 2 million adverse drug reactions (ADRs) each year with 100,000 deaths. There are a number of reasons for this increase:

- Many more drugs are prescribed.
- The more drugs a patient takes, the more chance there is of an ADR. Taking three or four medicines dramatically increases the risk.

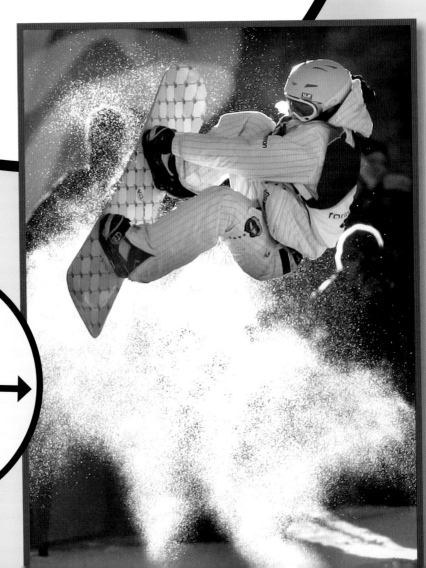

Extreme sports carry a risk and the snowboarder is aware of them. He believes that to him, the benefits – excitement, pleasure, satisfaction – outweigh the risks.

Reducing the risk

Animal testing is a key stage in the development of new medicines. There are strong arguments both for and against it.

Many people believe it is cruel to carry out experiments on animals. The thalidomide disaster is often used as an argument against animal testing. Thalidomide was shown to be safe in animals. However, it was never tested on pregnant animals. Following the withdrawal of thalidomide, there was a tightening up of drug testing regulations. All new drugs must now be tested extensively on animals.

Animal testing determines whether a drug is non-toxic, whether it is absorbed into the blood, and whether it reaches the right part of the body. It can also reveal how the drug is broken down by the body and how it is excreted. Unfortunately, animal testing cannot predict perfectly what will happen when humans take the drug. Some drugs have been non-toxic in animals but harmful to humans. However, animal testing does reduce the risk to human volunteers at the next stage of the process.

The use of animals in medical research is tightly controlled. The research establishment and a senior person at the site hold a licence. Every experiment must also be licensed. Inspectors visit regularly to check on conditions and the welfare of the animals.

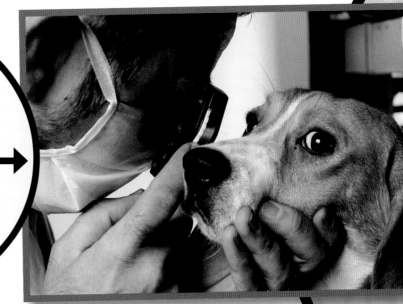

The three Rs

When working with animals, researchers follow three principles known as the three Rs:

- Reduce the number of experiments done on animals as much as possible.
- Replace animals with other testing techniques, such as computer modelling, wherever possible.
- Refine procedures when animals have to be used to minimize any suffering.

More medicines needed

Humans have an enemy that can make them seriously ill – a human cell that grows out of control. This is known as cancer. It occurs because the DNA of a cell is changed. This might be caused by ultraviolet light from the sun, radioactivity, chemicals, or even substances in our food. Some people's genes can make them more likely to develop particular types of cancer.

If the part of DNA that controls growth and replication is affected, the cell might multiply uncontrollably. The cells grow into a lump of many millions of cells called a **tumour**. Some tumours spread cells through the blood and lymph vessels to other parts of the body where new tumours grow. These tumours are described as **malignant**.

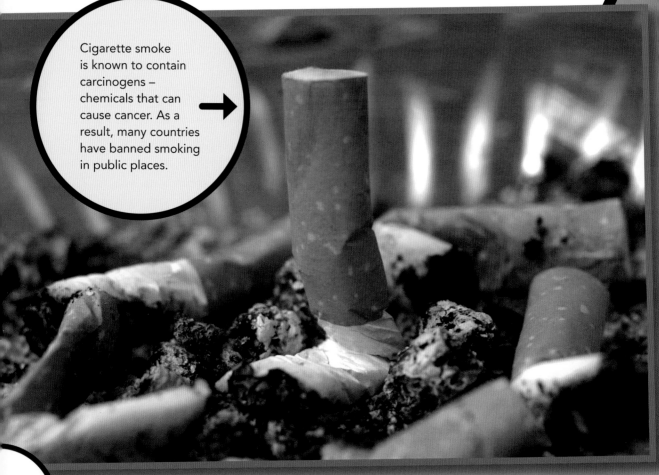

Cigarette smoke is known to contain carcinogens – chemicals that can cause cancer. As a result, many countries have banned smoking in public places.

Tackling cancer

For the last 50 years, cancer has been tackled in three main ways. If the tumour is caught early or is benign (not the type of tumour to spread through the body), it can be cut out. Secondly, **radiation** can be targeted at the cancer cells to kill them. Thirdly, chemicals can be used to kill rapidly dividing cells. This is called chemotherapy. It also kills other rapidly dividing cells in the bone marrow, reproductive system, and hair follicles. For this reason, people undergoing chemotherapy often lose their hair.

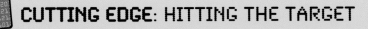

CUTTING EDGE: HITTING THE TARGET

New medicines are becoming available that are more specifically targeted against cancer cells. One approach is to help the body's natural immune system to recognize and destroy cancer cells. New treatments therefore include vaccines and substances that boost the immune system. Monoclonal antibodies (see below) target the antigens on cancer cells and other drugs cut off the blood supply to tumours.

Monoclonal antibodies

Medicines are usually small molecules. The pharmaceutical industry is much less keen on using large molecules such as proteins. Proteins cannot be taken as pills because they are digested in the stomach. They also "denature", which means they change shape and stop working. On the other hand, the body uses proteins for most of its important jobs and they are very versatile (have many uses).

A critical stage of drug development is finding a molecule that will bind specifically to its target. Nature is several steps ahead of us and has already created protein molecules that are highly specific – antibodies. Today, scientists are able to clone (make copies of) antibodies to recognize any structure. These monoclonal antibodies are a new type of medicine and they can be used to tackle cancer cells. Cancer cells have mutated (changed) receptors on their surface. Antibodies can be designed to recognize and attack them. The drug trastuzumab (Herceptin®), for example, recognizes a receptor on breast cancer cells. Monoclonal antibodies can also be used to carry toxic drugs or radioactive atoms to tumours to help destroy the cells.

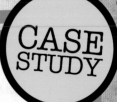

Penelope London

In 2007, Penelope London, a four-year-old American girl died after being refused a potentially life-saving treatment. Penelope suffered from a rare cancer of the nervous system. She was diagnosed with the cancer when she was just 16 months old. Doctors gave her only a 25 percent chance of being cured. In the following three years she received chemotherapy, radiation, bone marrow transplant, and surgery. She also tried some experimental therapies. As a result of all the treatment, Penelope stayed alive.

In late 2006, the cancer returned and no treatment would slow its progress. Penelope's father heard of a pharmaceutical company that was developing a new drug. The drug used a virus that normally affects pigs. When put in a human body, it seemed to attack certain cancer cells. The drug had only ever been given to six humans. The first patient treated with it had died – from cancer not the drug – and as a result further trials had been put on hold.

Penelope's parents asked the pharmaceutical company to make the drug available to their daughter. After many board meetings, the company refused. The company was concerned about the long-term prospects of their drug. If Penelope had been treated with it and still died, the trials might have been delayed for longer. Did Penelope have a right to try the experimental medicine? Was the company right to protect itself and the future of the drug for other patients, rather than trying to save Penelope?

Heart disease

The biggest killer in MEDCs is heart disease. Any disease that affects the heart, veins, and arteries is called a **cardiovascular** disease. The main cause of heart problems is the build up of **cholesterol**. This fatty material becomes deposited in the arteries and restricts blood flow. If the blockage prevents blood reaching the heart it can cause a heart attack.

High cholesterol levels can be caused by eating a fatty diet. Medicines called **statins** can reduce cholesterol. However, scientists have found that there are two types of cholesterol – good and bad. It is the balance between the two that is important. Now scientists are trying to develop medicines that contain a statin to reduce the bad cholesterol, and another drug to raise the good cholesterol.

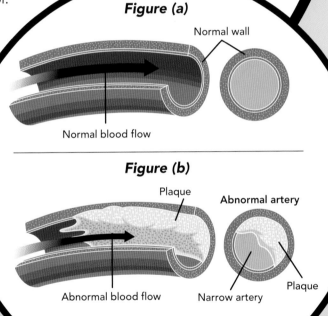

Figure (a)

Normal wall

Normal blood flow

Figure (a) shows a normal artery with normal blood flow. Figure (b) shows an artery with cholesterol build-up. A good diet and exercise avoids this problem but for some people it is not diagnosed until they have had a stroke or heart attack.

Figure (b)

Plaque

Abnormal artery

Abnormal blood flow

Narrow artery

Plaque

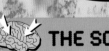

THE SCIENCE YOU LEARN: REDUCING CHOLESTEROL

Although there are drugs to treat high cholesterol, it is much better if people eat carefully. Foods such as eggs and prawns contain bad cholesterol. People with high cholesterol levels in their blood should avoid these foods. Foods that are high in saturated fats, such as butter, hard cheese, and fatty meat, raise cholesterol. On the other hand, fats described as unsaturated actually help to lower cholesterol levels. Foods high in unsaturated fats include oily fish, vegetable oils, nuts, and seeds. We should try to replace the saturated fats we eat with foods that contain unsaturated fats.

Diabetes – a growing problem

Diabetes is a condition in which the amount of glucose (sugar) in the blood is too high. A hormone called insulin is needed for the body to use glucose to provide energy. There are two main types of diabetes:

- Type 1 occurs when the body is unable to produce any insulin.
- Type 2 develops when the body can still make some insulin but not enough. Often this condition is linked with being overweight.

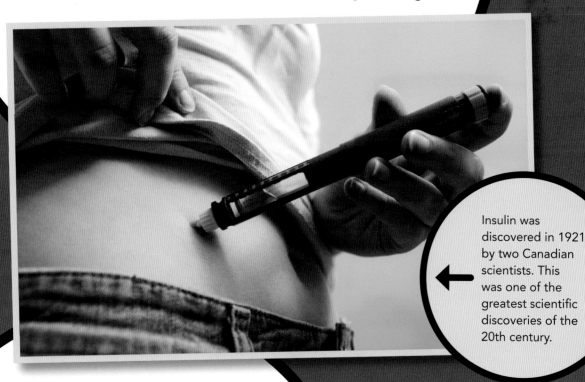

Insulin was discovered in 1921 by two Canadian scientists. This was one of the greatest scientific discoveries of the 20th century.

Treating diabetes

Diabetics need more insulin. There are two main ways to treat diabetes:

- Take drugs that either encourage the pancreas to make more insulin or assist the body in using its insulin more effectively.
- Inject insulin straight into the bloodstream. Many diabetics have to test their blood glucose level regularly and inject insulin if the glucose level is too high.

CUTTING EDGE: MAKING INSULIN

In the past, insulin was obtained from the pancreases of slaughtered animals such as pigs and sheep. Then scientists found the gene in human DNA that contained the instructions for making insulin. They made a copy of this gene and managed to insert it into the DNA of a bacterium. This strain of bacteria produces human insulin.

The modern epidemic

New medicines are curing many illnesses and life expectancy in MEDCs has increased significantly. However, there is one medical problem that is getting worse – obesity (excessive weight). Between 1995 and 2005, obesity rates in British men rose by 75 percent and in women by more than 50 percent. In the United States it is estimated that 40 million people are obese. Obesity can cause heart disease and type 2 diabetes. In the United States between 1990 and 2007, the number of diabetics rose by 76 percent.

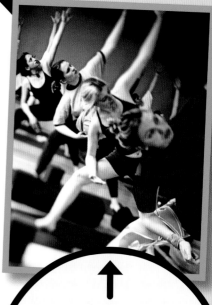

Body mass index (BMI)

BMI is a measure of weight relative to height. It is calculated by dividing mass in kilograms by height in metres squared. A person who is 1.7 m tall and weighs 85 kg has a BMI of $85/(1.7)^2 = 29.4$

The World Heath Organization (**WHO**) defines the following categories for BMI:

Underweight: <18.5
Normal: 18.5–24.9
Overweight: 25.0–29.9

Obesity: 30.0–39.9
Extreme obesity: >40

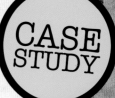

For most people, a healthy lifestyle involving a balanced diet and exercise will maintain body weight at the right level. Is it right to produce drugs to treat the excesses of modern life?

Are drugs the answer?

A large pharmaceutical company has now developed a drug to treat obesity. Researchers found that people who smoke the illegal drug cannabis often get ravenously hungry. The cannabis stimulates protein receptors in the brain and causes feelings of hunger. The company developed a drug that binds to the receptors and stops their action.

In 2006, the drug was approved for use in Europe, but approval was delayed in the United States. Blocking brain receptors that give feelings of pleasure, relaxation, and pain tolerance has a downside. People who took part in the drug trials showed anxiety, depression, and even suicidal thoughts.

CASE STUDY

Malaria – it takes just one bite

A parasite called *Plasmodium* causes the disease malaria. *Plasmodium* is carried by a certain type of female mosquito. If you are bitten by an infected mosquito, the parasite passes into your bloodstream. It travels to the liver where it grows and develops before passing back into the blood. It attacks red blood cells, causing aches and general weakness. After a few days, the person will have a high temperature, vomiting, a severe headache, and the shivers. It can be a fatal disease. Those that survive often never fully recover as the illness can return repeatedly.

Fighting malaria

There are two ways of fighting malaria. Drugs such as quinine kill the parasite in the bloodstream. Additionally there have been huge projects to eliminate the dangerous mosquito. Unfortunately, the parasite has become resistant to some of the drugs, and people have stopped taking precautions against the mosquito.

A sick child is treated for malaria. Killing the mosquitoes and clearing the wet places where they breed is important in the fight against the disease.

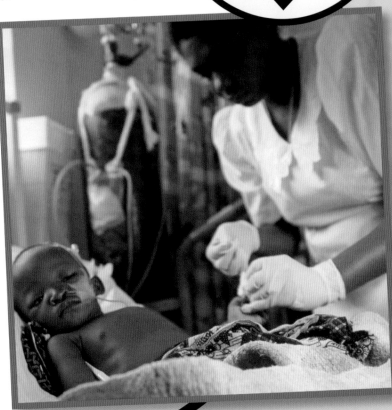

CUTTING EDGE: A VACCINE FOR MALARIA?

It is difficult to find a vaccine for malaria because the parasite hides itself inside red blood cells. However, two different methods are being trialled. In one, a section of DNA is used. The DNA carries the code for chemicals in the parasite that trigger an immune response. The DNA is injected into the patient. The human body takes up the DNA and makes the antigen. The alternative approach uses a weakened virus that has been genetically modified. The virus cannot reproduce in a human but will trigger an immune response.

Neglected diseases

Some diseases are disabling or life-threatening, but no treatments exist for them. Little research is carried out into them because the market for new medicines is too small to justify investment. These neglected diseases tend to occur in less-economically developed, tropical countries that cannot afford expensive medicines for millions of people.

- *Schistosomiasis (bilharzia)*. A parasitic disease caused by a flatworm. It can cause liver and intestinal damage. More than 200 million people are infected.
- *Lymphatic filariasis*. A parasitic disease caused by a microscopic worm. It causes chronic suffering, disability, and grotesquely swollen limbs (elephantiasis). Around 120 million people are infected.
- *Blinding trachoma*. An eye infection that can cause the eyelid to turn inward. The eye lashes rub on the eyeball resulting in intense pain, scarring, and blindness. Around 80 million people are infected.
- *Onchocerciasis (river blindness)*. This is caused by a parasitic worm transmitted by a fly. It causes severe skin disease, visual impairment, blindness, and shortened life expectancy. Around 37 million people are infected.
- *Chagas' disease*. This tropical parasitic disease is passed to humans by a blood-sucking insect. If untreated, the disease is fatal. Between 16 million and 18 million people are infected.
- *Leishmaniasis*. This disease is caused by a parasite transmitted by a tiny sandfly. One form of the disease leads to ulcers and permanent scarring. Another form destroys the mucous membranes in the nose, mouth, and throat causing horrendous disfigurement. More than 12 million people are infected.

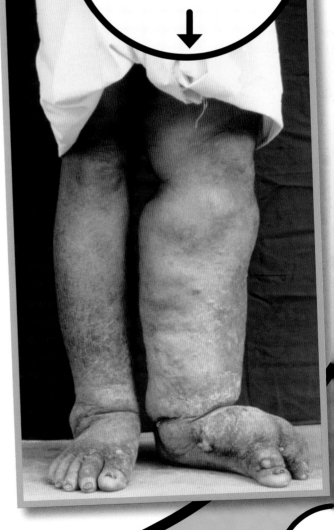

The disease elephantiasis causes the tissue in the skin to swell. Research into neglected diseases like this one is largely funded by charities. Most sufferers do not live in countries that can afford new drugs.

The future – issues and challenges

In the quest for new medicines, scientists are searching for natural products that will treat some of our most dangerous diseases. Pharmaceutical companies are hunting for life-saving chemicals in plants, animals, fungi, and bacteria. Many existing drugs were originally derived from natural sources. The breast cancer drug, taxol, was developed from the bark of the Pacific yew tree. Aggrastat, a drug that prevents blood clotting, came from the venom of the African saw-scaled viper.

Is borrowing from nature a good thing? It encourages people to maintain the wide diversity of living things on our planet. Large pharmaceutical companies also benefit, but the local people gain nothing. This has been called biopiracy.

Alternatives to medicines

When we are ill, we usually reach for a packet of pills. Some people argue that instead of giving pills to hyperactive children or to depressed adults, for example, we should encourage them to diet and exercise. Increasingly, people want pills to help them cope with the demands of modern lifestyles. Are we too quick to reach for the medicine bottle?

CUTTING EDGE: PHARMING

The joining of farming and pharmaceuticals is called **pharming**. A range of farm animals have been genetically engineered to produce useful medicines. To get the new medicine, the animal is simply milked. A blood clotting agent has been produced in sheep's milk in this way, and cows have been modified to produce a protein used to treat traumatic injuries. The animals can end up with birth defects and may age prematurely.

Some people feel that it is wrong to modify animals in this way and that animals should be treated with more respect. Others feel that the benefits to human health are more important.

Those who eat a balanced diet and stay fit are likely to suffer less from illnesses that require medicines. To try and keep healthy, we should eat less saturated fat and eat plenty of fruit and vegetables for their fibre and valuable antioxidant chemicals. We know that some fish oils are good for the brain. We also know that exercise is good for us, both physically and mentally.

Modern Chinese medicine

While most of the world wants access to modern medicines, there is an alternative medical system. Chinese herbal medicine goes back to the 3rd century BC.

The traditional use of plant remedies is often based on the biological effects of the chemicals in them. The natural chemicals in plants are more complex than modern pharmaceuticals, and because Chinese medicine usually involves a mixture of herbs, the components balance each other. As a result, side effects are rare and such medicines are claimed to be both effective and safe. Chinese medicines are also designed to treat internal imbalances in the body rather than symptoms alone.

Modern Chinese herbal medicine is combined with acupuncture, dietary therapy, and exercises in movement and breathing to treat the whole person. Many illnesses are treated successfully in this way.

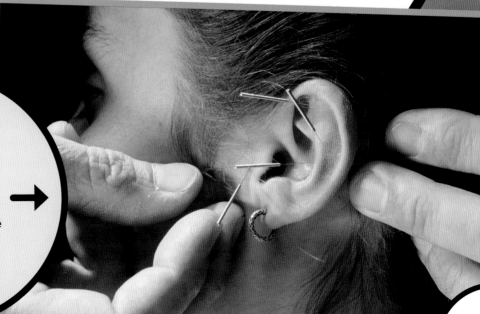

Acupuncture originated about 3,000 years ago in China. Now that western scientists know more about the control of pain, they realize that acupuncture might stimulate the production of natural painkillers in the body.

The cost of drugs

Many governments and health agencies are concerned about the cost of medicines. The amount spent on drugs rises each year. In the United Kingdom, the amount spent on drugs rose by 40 percent between 2000 and 2004. In the United States, almost half the population uses a prescription drug, and the amount spent on them has risen by 15 percent in each of the past 20 years.

In countries where patients pay only small prescription charges, some authorities restrict which medicines can be prescribed. In countries where health insurance covers the cost, insurance premiums have risen to a level that people cannot always afford.

Price controls

In some countries, government agencies work with pharmaceutical companies to set the price of medicines. This can keep the cost down. In the United States there is no regulation and prices are higher. American citizens are often tempted to visit Canada or Mexico where drugs are much cheaper, even though it is illegal to do so.

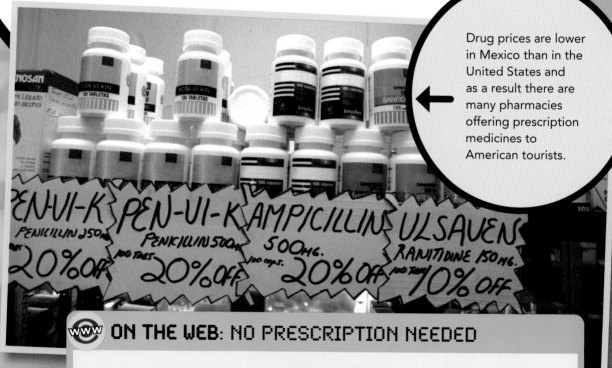

Drug prices are lower in Mexico than in the United States and as a result there are many pharmacies offering prescription medicines to American tourists.

www **ON THE WEB**: NO PRESCRIPTION NEEDED

Many prescription medicines can be bought on the Internet. The price is always cheaper, but there are risks. The patient does not see a doctor and the drug could be dangerous for them. The drug could even be a fake or contain harmful chemicals.

Helping LEDCs

As a result of improved living conditions, better healthcare, and good medicines, life expectancy in more economically developed countries (MEDCs) has increased significantly. However, many people in LEDCs have always struggled to afford medicines. The problem is particularly bad when new medicines are still under patent, and therefore very expensive. In 2006, the WHO criticized big pharmaceutical companies. It said that people were dying because they could not gain access to affordable life-saving medicines. In response, the pharmaceutical companies say they will give the medicines free or at low prices, but that the LEDCs lack the ability to distribute and prescribe the medicines correctly.

A new model

As you read on page 41, there are many diseases which affect LEDCs that have few medicines available to treat them. When drugs do exist, they are often too expensive. Recently there have been new efforts to address this problem. Partnerships have been set up in which pharmaceutical companies work with charities to develop new medicines for neglected diseases.

CASE STUDY

Aid for Africa

In recent years, some large pharmaceutical companies have increased their donations to Africa. In 2006, GlaxoSmithKline (GSK) gave U.S. $600 million to charitable initiatives, a large amount of which went to LEDCs in Africa. Since 1988, the company has donated 600 million treatments for elephantiasis. GSK also funds the Mobilizing for Malaria and Positive Action for HIV/AIDS initiatives that deliver education, prevention, and health care services in many African countries. The company also provides drugs to treat HIV/AIDS and malaria at no-profit for 64 countries in Africa. Other companies make similar donations but critics argue that they could do a lot more.

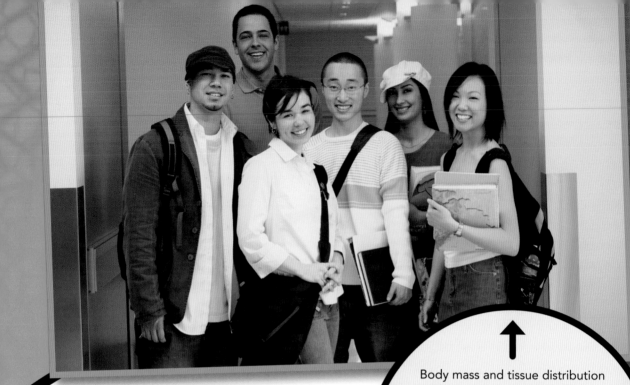

Body mass and tissue distribution differ in men and women. They might experience disease in different ways and respond to medicines differently. Ethnic differences might also lead to different responses. Understanding the genetics of each person would enable selective prescribing of medicines.

Personalized medicines

The pharmaceutical industry has traditionally produced medicines to target particular diseases. They are given to anyone suffering from the disease. This "one size fits all" approach is beginning to change. What works for one person might not be effective in another. As a better understanding of genetics and biological molecules develops, medicine is getting closer to developing more personalized drugs.

"His" and "hers" medicines

Some drugs that work on women do not necessarily work on men, and side effects might vary between the sexes. A few of the most significant differences include:

- Some painkillers work better in women than in men.
- Women suffer more severe reactions to certain HIV drugs.
- Lung cancer treatments work differently in each sex.
- One drug for bowel disease is only licensed for women.

However, we still do not know enough about sex differences and more research is needed.

Ethnic differences

Some diseases affect certain human groups more than others. Sickle cell disease is common in people of African-Caribbean origin. Type 2 diabetes is particularly common in people from southern Asia. While such observations are not controversial, suggesting that medicines could be targeted at particular ethnic groups is certain to cause intense debate.

Fantasy or the future – smart pills

If you could take a drug to boost your brain power, would you? Drugs to enhance performance are nothing new. Students have taken caffeine tablets to allow them to study through the night. Lorry drivers have been known to use amphetamines. Of course the use of such drugs is dangerous, and provides only temporary effects. However, a new type of brain enhancer can improve mental functions in a lasting way. Another drug sold for sleep disorders is proving popular amongst healthy people who want to improve their thinking power.

Where will it stop? Is it acceptable for parents to give their children brain-enhancing drugs? Will educational success in the future depend upon access to the latest drugs?

 CUTTING EDGE: WIPE AWAY THE PAIN?

Scientists have now discovered a drug that can dull the pain of traumatic events. Called propranolol, the drug was originally developed to treat high blood pressure. Doctors noticed that patients using it suffered fewer signs of stress when recalling a trauma. The drug disrupts the way memories are stored. This could help people suffering from real trauma, but it is also open to abuse. Healthy people might try to block out memories of embarrassing behaviour or failed relationships.

Balance it all up

There is no doubt that medicines have benefited mankind tremendously. Some diseases that were once rampant have been all but eliminated. New treatments are tackling illnesses that were considered incurable. However, there are many issues involved in the discovery, development, and delivery of new drugs. Debate will continue over many of them.

Facts and figures

Some leading figures in drug development

Li Shi Chen

Chinese author and highly influential figure in Chinese medicine, Li Shi Chen (1518-93) wrote the famous *Great Compendium of Herbs*. Li Shi Chen's grandfather and father were physicians, but he was encouraged to study literature. However, as a boy he was frequently ill, and this drove him to become a doctor. Li Shi Chen studied hard and by the age of 27 was respected for his medical abilities. He continued to read all he could on medicine but found many contradictions, errors, and irrelevancies in the books. At the age of 30 he began to write his own book. It took him another 30 years to complete his great work, which sadly was only published after his death.

Henry Wellcome

Born in a log cabin in Wisconsin, USA, Henry Wellcome (1853–1936) was the son of a travelling missionary. Henry had an early interest in medicine and in 1880 he and a partner founded Burroughs Wellcome & Company, selling medicines to England. Up to that time, medicines had mainly been sold as powders. Wellcome invented the pill form of medicine. When Burroughs died, Wellcome set up several research laboratories. In 1910, he became a British citizen and before long set up the Wellcome Foundation. After he died his wealth was used to set up the Wellcome Trust, the world's largest private biomedical charity.

Howard Florey

Australian scientist Howard Florey (1898–1968) was brought up in Adelaide, Australia at the beginning of the 20th century. Florey won a scholarship to Oxford University in England. There he eventually became Professor of Pathology. In 1938 while researching into antibacterial chemicals he began to look again at penicillin, discovered 10 years earlier. Fleming had extracted penicillin from mould but not in a concentrated form. However in 1939 in collaboration with Ernst Chain, Florey managed to manufacture and purify a small amount of the drug. It still took time to scale up the process to manufacture large quantities but in 1945 Florey, Chain, and Fleming were jointly awarded the Nobel Prize for Medicine.

Frances Kelsey

Canadian pharmacologist Frances Kelsey (born 1914) graduated from McGill University, Canada, and went to the University of Chicago, USA, to help set up a new pharmacology department. In 1960, Kelsey was hired by the FDA and asked to review a new drug, thalidomide. It had already been approved in more than 20 European and African countries, but Kelsey withheld approval for it. Despite pressure from thalidomide's manufacturer, Kelsey persisted in requesting information to explain a report of a nervous system side effect. Soon the horrific side effects of thalidomide became apparent and Kelsey was regarded as a heroine for saving the United States from a tragedy.

Sir James Black

James Black (born in Scotland in 1924) worked as a doctor, a university academic, and in the pharmaceutical industry. He is most famous for his invention of propranolol, a treatment for high blood pressure and angina (a painful heart complaint). Its discovery is considered to be one of the most important contributions to medicine in the 20th century. Black also synthesized cimetidine, a drug that stops the stomach producing too much acid. In 1988, he was awarded the Nobel Prize for Medicine.

Bill Gates

Former chairman of Microscoft, American businessman Bill Gates (born 1955) is the world's richest man. In 2000, he and his wife Melinda (born 1965) set up a charitable foundation with a donation of U.S. $126 million. The Bill and Melinda Gates Foundation gives grants to the Global Health Program, investing in research into treatments for HIV and neglected diseases. It also aims to bring together people with expertise in treating malaria in a drive to eliminate the disease.

Top 10 causes of death in high and low income countries

High income countries		Low income countries	
Disease	**Percentage of deaths**	**Disease**	**Percentage of deaths**
Coronary heart disease	17.1	Coronary heart disease	10.8
Stroke and other cerebrovascular (brain blood vessel) diseases	9.8	Lower respiratory infections	10
Windpipe and lung cancers	5.8	HIV/AIDS	7.5
Lower respiratory (lung) infections	4.3	Complications at birth	6.4
Chronic obstructive pulmonary disease (type of lung disease)	3.9	Stroke and other cerebrovascular diseases	6
Colon and rectum (bowel) cancers	3.3	Diarrhoeal diseases	5.4
Alzheimer's and other dementias	2.7	Malaria	4.4
Type 2 diabetes	2.7	Tuberculosis	3.8
Breast cancer	1.9	Chronic obstructive pulmonary disease	3.1
Stomach cancer	1.8	Road traffic accidents	1.9

(Source: The World Health Organization http://www.who.int/mediacentre/factsheets/fs310/en/index.html)

Top 10 blockbuster drugs

"Blockbusters" are drugs for common diseases that generate millions (even billions) of pounds in profits. Pharmaceutical companies are always looking for a new blockbuster.

Trade name	Generic name	Annual sales (£ billion)	Maker	Condition treated
Lipitor®	atorvastatin	6.9	Pfizer	High cholesterol
Nexium®	esomeprazole	3.4	AstraZeneca	Heartburn
Seretide/ Advair®	fluticasone/ salmeterol	3.1	GlaxoSmithKline	Asthma
Plavix®	clopidogrel	2.9	Bristol-Myers Squibb	Heart disease
Norvasc®	amlodipine	2.5	Pfizer	Hypertension
Aranesp®	darbepoetin alfa	2.5	Amgen	Anaemia
Zyprexa®	olanzapine	2.3	Eli Lilly	Bipolar disorder (depression)
Risperdal®	risperidone	2.3	Johnson & Johnson	Schizophrenia
Embrel®	etanercept	2.2	Amgen/Wyeth	Arthritis
Effexor®	venlafaxine	2.0	Wyeth	Depression

(Source: The UK Pharmaceutical Directory www.pharmaceutical.org.uk/pharmaceutical-product/index.html This list was compiled in 2006. Track changes in it by searching for the Top 10 Blockbuster Prescription Drugs.)

Top 10 incurable diseases

Modern medicine has done much to eradicate and cure disease, but it has failed in some areas. One disease that is yet to be cured is suffered by millions of people in the world every year – the common cold.

Disease	Description
Ebola	A fatal viral infection that causes high fever and internal bleeding.
Polio	A viral infection that has been virtually eliminated as a result of vaccinations. There is still no cure for anyone not protected.
Lupus erythematosus	Simply known as lupus, this is an autoimmune disease that causes inflammation in various parts of the body.
Influenza	Also known as the flu it is a viral infection of the upper or lower respiratory tract (windpipe and lungs) that is marked by fever and chills.
Creutzfeldt-Jakob disease (CJD)	A rare degenerative disease of the central nervous system. Usually fatal within one year.
Diabetes	An inability of the body to produce or respond to insulin and maintain proper levels of glucose in the blood.
AIDS	Acquired immunodeficiency syndrome – a disease of the immune system caused by the human immunodeficiency virus (HIV).
Asthma	A disorder of the lungs in which inflamed airways are constricted, causing breathlessness, wheezing, and coughing.
Cancer	A group of more than 100 distinct diseases in which there is uncontrolled growth of abnormal cells in the body.
Common cold	A viral infection that starts in the upper respiratory tract and may cause secondary infections in the eyes or middle ears.

(Source: The List Universe http://listverse.com/health/top-10-incurable-diseases)

Find out more

The story of medicine and our needs for new treatments is a fascinating one. This book can only give you a brief introduction to the topic. Many issues have only been touched on or not covered at all. Find out more by using the sources below.

Further reading

Anderson, Judith. *Working For Our Future: Fighting Disease* (Franklin Watts, 2007)

Arnold, Nick. *Horrible Science: Measly Medicine* (Scholastic, 2006)

Tames, Richard. *Turning Points in History: Penicillin* (2nd ed.) (Heinemann Library, 2006)

Townsend, John. *A Painful History of Medicine: Pills, Powders & Potions* (Raintree, 2008)

Websites

http://ahha.org/rosen.htm
Learn about the holistic approach to healthcare.

http://commtechlab.msu.edu/sites/dlc-me/zoo
Visit the microbe zoo to learn more about how we rely on bacteria and fungi.

www.abpi-careers.org.uk
Find out about careers in the pharmaceutical industry.

www.bbc.co.uk/health
Find information on many diseases as well as how to live a healthy lifestyle.

www.botany.hawaii.edu/faculty/wong/BOT135/Lect21b.htm
Discover all there is to know about penicillin.

www.cellsalive.com/howbig.htm
See how the sizes of bacteria and viruses compare and find out all about the immune system and microbiology.

www.wellcome.ac.uk
Find out more about the work of the Wellcome Foundation.

www.historylearningsite.co.uk/history_of_medicine.htm
Explore this site for a comprehensive history of early medicine used by the Egyptians, ancient Greeks, and Romans.

www.kidshealth.org/teen/diseases_conditions/allergies_immune/allergies.html
In an allergic reaction the body's immune system turns on itself. Find out more on the kids' health website.

www.pbs.org/opb/intimatestrangers/index.html
Find out why microbes are so important to life on Earth.

www.thevaccinesite.org
This site gives you a good introduction to how vaccinations work and the diseases you may be vaccinated against.

www.who.int/topics/infectious_diseases/en
Discover more about infectious diseases from the World Health Organization website.

www.stopanimaltests.org/index.aspx and **www.abpi.org.uk/amric/amric.asp**
Explore both sides of the animal testing debate.

Glossary

AIDS   disease in which the body's natural defence against infection is destroyed.

antibiotic   chemical that prevents the growth of or kills microorganisms such as bacteria, fungi, and parasites

antibody   protein that is used by the immune system to identify and destroy cells or organisms that should not be in the body

antigen   chemical on the surface of an invading cell or virus that triggers a response from the immune system

bacterium   single-celled microorganism (plural, bacteria)

cardiovascular   relating to the heart and blood vessels

cholesterol   fat-like material that the body naturally makes and is found in some food stuffs

clinical trial   test of a new medical treatment comparing it with existing treatments or a placebo

cyclooxygenase   type of enzyme that is responsible for the formation of chemicals called prostaglandins

DNA   (deoxyribonucleic acid) contains the instructions for the growth and function of all living things

drug candidate   chemical that has the potential to become a medicine

enzyme   protein that catalyses (speeds up) a chemical reaction in living things

foetus   unborn baby in its mother's womb

fungus   class of living things more closely related to animals than plants; includes yeasts, moulds, and mushrooms

gene   section of DNA that carries the instruction for a particular characteristic

generic   not having a brand name

HIV   human immunodeficiency virus which causes AIDS

immune system   mechanisms in an organism that protect against disease by killing pathogens (disease-producing agents) and tumour cells

macrophage   type of white blood cell that engulfs and digests pathogens

malignant   type of tumour that is cancerous

microbe   organism such as a virus, bacterium, or fungus that can only be seen under a microscope

monoclonal antibody   antibodies that are all identical because they have been produced by one type of immune cell. They are designed to recognize particular antigens.

parasite   plant or animal that lives on or in another, usually larger, host organism in a way that harms or is of no advantage to the host

patent   exclusive right officially granted by a government to an inventor to make or sell an invention. No other person or organization can make or market the invention.

pharmaceutical   drug used in medicine

pharming   production of medically valuable proteins from genetically modified animals and plants

placebo   dummy medicine containing no active ingredient that is given to some patients in a clinical trial. Its effect is compared to the new drug being trialled.

prostaglandin   substance produced throughout the body that is involved in inflammation and pain messages

protein   large complicated chemical that makes cells the size and shape they are

radiation   type of energy wave, used in radiotherapy to treat cancer

receptor   protein molecule embedded in a cell membrane. Receptors receive messages from other cells. When a messenger molecule binds onto a receptor, chemical signals travel rapidly to the nucleus.

side effect   unintended result of taking a drug

soluble   able to be dissolved. Sugar is soluble in water.

statin   type of drug used to lower cholesterol levels

tumour   lump of cancerous cells

vaccine   liquid containing microbes, their parts, or products used to control disease by making people immune

virus   microscopic infectious agent that is unable to grow or reproduce outside a cell of another organism

World Health Organization (WHO)   agency concerned with setting standards of public health, and monitoring and tackling infectious diseases throughout the world

Index